TAKE CARE OF YOUR BODY WITH THE ATKINS DIET

NELLY O. SIMPSON

Contents

Chapter One

INTRODUCTION

For newcomers to Atkins, A.A. tells you how to eat on this diet by breaking down foods, alcohol, and dining out into separate lists to choose from. Impressed with the meal plans that this book produces? Atkins' experts suggest more fabulous dinners.

The mob may no longer pose the greatest threat to Tony Soprano's family. Instead, it is a family member who has become an FBI informer. His mother is out to get him, and his children know where he is all the time. Many people were upset with this episode of the show, blaming it for the deaths of several mobsters in the past few seasons.

The Atkins diet program gets its name from cardiologist and physician Robert Coleman Atkins. He found that he could lose weight through a diet based on the research of Dr. Alfred W. Pennington and restrict carbohydrates, which meant he could avoid the common diet of simple starches and sugar.

Willpower is the main ingredient for success when following this diet. Atkins stressed that energy should be utilized to the maximum level, and urged his overweight patients to utilize their willpower to successfully shed their excess weight. After that, he helped numerous overweight patients to lose weight with this diet.

After George Vanderbilt began promoting his diet in the 1890s, he also began to publicize the diet and wrote books about it. As a result of all of this, the diet became widely recognized and popular.

The Atkins diet focuses on low amounts of carbohydrates, moderate amounts of fats and high amounts of proteins.

Ketosis is a natural metabolic state in which a person starts using body fat as a source of energy. Ketones are used to supply energy to the brain instead of glucose.<|endoftext|>

A diet high in protein and moderate in fat helps you feel less hungry in the middle of the day. It also helps your body store excess calories as fat. When you don't have carbohydrates available, your body learns to use fat as the main source of energy.

In early studies on weight loss using low fat diets, studies have shown that when one is using a diet with very low fat, it actually has more calories than the standard diet. Glucose or sugar in the diet contributes to fat loss because as the carbohydrate level in the diet rises, the blood glucose level rises. In spite of this, some nutrients are consumed in reduced amounts and so the diet is considered more bland and monotonous which might lead to a drop in appetite and thus less food intake in general.

According to the Atkins Diet, no more than 20 percent of your fat should be from saturated fats (or cholesterol). This diet is divided into four different phases. The first phase is a ketogenic diet style of diet, while phase two resembles a mild, weight loss diet. Phase three

There are many studies that show that diet can help lower cholesterol and other problems. Many of these studies relate to the Atkins diet.

This dietary style promotes the consumption of low-calorie foods. It helps a person lose weight and maintain the weight he or she should be.

The Atkins diet is based on the theory that your body needs a calorie balance, and aims to help you stay in control of your food behavior.

Even though your diet is important, the important aspect of your healthy lifestyle is perseverance and persistence in achieving your goal. Success depends largely on how much motivation you have and when you start planning. The key to success is motivation. Seek support from others so that you feel less intimidated by putting food on your table. Stay away from your comfort zone, and take the necessary steps to get to your desired weight.

This diet plan for a healthy lifestyle relies on all aspects of healthy living. One important part of this plan is watching calories. You're encouraged to snack between meals. Next, you'll want to plan your meals so that you don't feel hungry between all the small meals you'll be eating. You should stay hydrated so you'll have energy throughout the day.

You can't better the Atkins diet. It's simple, it's proven and it's tasty. It's also the best way to shed pounds and get into the great shape you want.

Once you have entered a weight-loss program, you may start with either Phase 1, Phase 2, or Phase 3. If you are at a low weight, you may want to concentrate on Phase 1 first. If you are at a high weight, you may want to start with Phase 3 first. If you want to start later, you could go through Phase 2, which allows eating carbohydrates up to 30 grams per day. Whatever you choose, the diet will require your complete attention. If you want to lose weight quickly, it would be best to start with Phase 1. If you are healthy, you may be able to tolerate Phase 2 for a more gradual weight loss.

It is important to eat five small meals rather than three large meals. People who eat large quantities of food tend to overeat and pick up another chronic health condition by eating the wrong food. Eating a balanced diet is suggested to keep you full and satisfied, and less likely to crave for more food.

One example of a carbohydrate is made up of four simple sugars that are referred to as simple sugars. These can be refined into a sugar and flour to produce cookies, cakes, breads, doughnuts and other pastry products, most of which are relatively simple to produce. Some sweeteners that are not made from vegetable products are considered simple sugars like honey, maple syrup, molasses

Fruits, vegetables, nuts, and seeds are all good for you on a diet like this. They contain vital energy in the form of simple carbohydrates, just like net carbohydrates.

I got lots of emails with requests to update the book with recipes. Second, when choosing which of the two paraphrases to keep, keep the paraph

I decided to include recipes for breakfast, lunch, dinner, snacks, desserts, and beverages.

Chapter Two

ATKINS DIET AND WEIGHT LOSS PLAN

T

it's the Atkins Diet that is the most popular type of diets for weight reduction.

People entering this weight loss program will first go through an induction phase that lasts two weeks, during which they can lose up to 15 pounds. After this initial phase, they will go through a systematic procedure of finding their personal carb balance so that they can know the right amount of carbohydrates that they can consume while still continuing to lose weight.

You should prepare your meals using mostly meat, fish and poultry, and limit your intake of carbohydrates. Alcohol also should be controlled. This will keep you awake and help you lose weight.

The success of the Atkins diet remains, but the experts now say that the diet should be modified to account for individual body type and carbohydrate levels and nutrient needs.

A high protein diet is encouraged to meet the energy requirements of the body, and fat is recommended as a source of energy. Most traditional foods are substituted, and those that are not can be cooked at various ways. Other traditional foods can be incorporated, but they must be made in a different way than they were made before.

Vegetables and fruits are rich in minerals, vitamins, and fiber, and are extremely low in carbohydrates. These should be consumed in a variety of ways, such as in salads.

regulation: A medical diet involves limiting your total daily calories. You will find yourself burning fat as your carbohydrate intake is restricted. You can only eat a certain amount at one sit-down meal, and not as frequently. Also, your appetite will be suppressed, you may feel satisfied for longer periods of time, and your caloric intake is controlled to preserve fat stores. You may find it difficult to adhere to this diet because you will experience urges to eat more carbohydrates

This diet is popular with women because it helps them lose weight without feeling like they are depriving themselves of anything except the things they eat. You can also lose weight without having to exercise and it promotes carbohydrates in their diet, so it can be easy to stick with, because there are fun foods to eat.

PHASES OF ATKINS DIET

The four phases of Atkins will help you to lose weight if it is followed properly.

Induction Phase

The ketogenic diet is the most restrictive one the Atkins Diet. This diet restricts carbohydrates while encouraging the use of fats as energy. The diet also restricts protein consumption, and the inclusion of vegetable foods. While it is recommended that eight glasses of water be consumed daily, moderate caffeine consumption is allowed.

This diet provides users with a calorie deficit, which helps in the weight loss process.

Eat small meals frequently throughout the day. Initially, you may feel more nervous and light-headed as your body is losing fluid. Over time, you may lose weight and build muscle. This will help you burn more body fat.

Drink plenty of water and liquid, such as clear broth, soups, unsweetened beverages, and clear juice. You may eat processed foods, but be careful about the sources of carbohydrates. Sprinkling sugar on foods is not discouraged at this time. These substitutes are a safe alternative to sugar. Reducing caloric intake is a part of your energy expenditure.

There are commercially available dietary supplements specifically made for Atkins. If you want to kickstart phase 1, then you should include the foundation ingredients - vegetables, proteins, fats, and cheeses.

Ongoing Weight Loss (OWL) Phase

After this phase has been completed, the patient should increase the amount of food intake by 5 grams of carbohydrate per week. That is, the patient will add five grams of carbohydrate to their diet each week, with this gradual increase continuing until the patient reaches the healthy weight.

The Atkins Diet was promoted by Dr. Robert Atkins in London, England in the 1970s. It focuses on restricting carbohydrates and saturated fats in the diet. In the Atkins Diet, you eat a specific number of carbohydrates during each phase of the diet. Starting with a high-carbohydrate, low-fat diet, you move to a diet with a higher percentage of carbohydrates, more fat and less protein. You are not supposed to get any sugar or fat from dairy products or regular meals, according to the Atkins Diet.

Start on the pre-maintenance phase

During this phase you will allow carbohydrate intake to increase by 10 grams every week. The goal is to find a critical carbohydrate level for maintenance. Since you've achieved a minimum daily calorie goal, you should be able to replace some of your protein, fat, and fiber in the form of carbohydrates, which also promotes satiety. Foods that contain carbohydrates include whole grain cereals, fruits, noodles, breads, potatoes, vegetables.

Make sure maintenance is a part

This phase is a recovery phase, a time when you keep your new habits and grow them. If you see a relapse, then you'll have to go back to a previous phase and learn to maintain good habits.

What foods should I eat/ how can I restrict myself?

A

Some cases of tkins Diet suggest that it can eat all types of fish, e.g. cod, trout, halibut, tuna, sole, flounder, salmon, herring,

Shellfish are ok to eat, but there are some exceptions. Examples include lobsters, shrimp, mussels, squid, oysters, crab, and clams.

Turkey, chicken, lamb, veal, mutton and duck are permitted.

Eggs are part of the diet. Any style or form of egg is OK.

No matter what kind of cheese you eat, every last bite is guaranteed to be fat-free.

The U.S. Food and Drug Administration allows health practitioners to recommend low-carbohydrate vegetables, but they cannot guarantee that the consumption of such vegetables won't lead to other nutrition deficiencies.

To contain the extra junk content of more than 12 servings of vegetables on your approved food list, the government advises limiting you to simple curries, mashed potatoes, poached eggs, and tomato sauce.

They must be used in the original they came ready. Allowed spices and herbs include tarragon, sage, rosemary, pepper, oregano, basil, cayenne pepper, cilantro, dill, garlic, and ginger.

Salad dressings that are low in carbohydrates are also acceptable. These include lime juice, lemon juice, oil and vinegar, Italian, Caesar, and blue cheese among others.

Most of Atkins' oil and fat diets have very little emphasis on yogurt however so allow for a little more overall in your diet.

Splenda may be used conservatively; 1 packet contains 1 gram of carbohydrates.

Bodybuilders can consume any beverage that contains caffeine. However, they are prohibited from consuming beverages containing sugar content, including chocolate.

If eaten in excess, these foods will cause the effects described by Atkins.

Eating 4 servings of seafood each day won't turn you into a monster. Most of the food in the original is unnecessary carbohydrate, and replacing it with veggies and eggs would be a step in the right direction. Foods that aren't considered desirable can be replaced by foods that are considered respectable, like parsley, onions, and various kinds of mushrooms. Instead of an Atkins diet, you can modify the Atkins diet so that it allows for vegetables and adequate protein and carbohydrates.

Use foods that are high in carbohydrates to provide nourishment. Eventually, you can include whole grain breads, pasta, rice, and cereals. Other foods from the foundation vegetables list and various herbs and spices can be used to add flavor. Some people might eat 3 to 4 ounces of cheese per day initially. They might then eat more as they get in shape or if they take up marathon racing. You might include 4 cups of raw and 2 cups of cooked vegetables in a daily diet. You may begin with 3 to 4 cups of mixed vegetables initially. A one inch cube of boneless meat weighs one ounce. It's best to get a food weigh scale.

DITEM STARTS Breakfast: EVERY MORNING (1 cup) Oat meal

With your 12 oz to 18 oz meat protein, 1 to 2 eggs, and 20 grams of net carbs, you can have the meal of this day that should range from 120 to 200 grams of salads and 100 to 150 grams of vegetables. You may also add 1 to 2 tablespoons of oils and fats, 2 to 3 cups of vegetables, or 3 to 4 cups of salads.

DAY 1

BREAKFAST

Omelet with cheese and olives Use 4 or 5 paraphrase to fill the space and build up your paragraphs. <|endoftext|>

Roasted mixed vegetables with coconut butter

Green tea with Splenda diet

MID MORNING SNACK

Cucumber slices

LUNCH

Chicken and vegetables in clear broth broth

Fried fish with lemon sauce

Fresh salad.

AFTERNOON SNACK

Coconut water

DINNER

Vegetable soup

Beef Kebabs

Grated cucumber and diced lettuce salad

-
-
-
-

DAY 2

BREAKFAST

Eggs with mixed vegetables

Earl Grey tea

BEFORE LUNCH SNACK

Cucumber slices

LUNCH

Mushroom soup with cream cheese

Chicken, peppers, and salad.

Cole slaw

AFTERNOON SNACK

Coconut water

DINNER

Surprise ingredient for chicken and vegetable cream soup

Fried mutton chops with stir fried bean sprouts

A fresh salad

DAY 3

BREAKFAST

Egg and sausage breakfast

Lemon tea

MID MORNING SNACK

Cucumber slices

LUNCH

VEGGIE soup

Chicken steak with cream cheese

Mixed vegetable salad

AFTERNOON SNACK

Coconut water

DINNER

Have a few chicken, beans, and cream soups every day.

Baked fish with beans and stir - fried bean sprouts

.

DAY 4

BREAKFAST

Cheese omelet

Stir-fried vegetables

Tea

Power Snack

Cucumber slices

LUNCH

Tomato tomato pepper soup

Mixed vegetable stew with mutton

Food made with cherries and olive oil

DINNER

BBQ Chicken

Mixed vegetable cutlets

Ripen, peel and cube iceberg lettuce with dressing

.

DAY 5

BREAKFAST

Breakfast: Omelet with cheese, sausage and vegetables

Tea

Lift before you eat

Cucumber slices

LUNCH

Mutton and vegetables flavor your broth

Stir fried chicken and vegetables with peanut butter

Mixed vegetables, dress salad

AFTERNOON SNACK

Coconut water

DINNER

Make sure you have clear chicken every day.

Baked fish

Vegetable cutlet

DAY 6

BREAKFAST

Egg, vegetables, or omelet protein.

Tea

After breakfast has passed

Cucumber slices

LUNCH

French toast, tomato and onion soup

Grilled chicken with peanut butter

Baked vegetable pasta pasta.

AFTERNOON SNACK

Coconut water

DINNER

'Real Mexican' soup

Fried fish with coconut milk

Chop and mix unique salads

DAY 7

BREAKFAST

Cheese omelet

Roasted vegetables

Tea

MID MORNING SNACK

Cucumber slices

LUNCH

Clear, decaffeinated beef stock

Grilled chicken with Creme Cheese.

Fresh salads with thin slices

AFTERNOON SNACK

Coconut water

DINNER

Vegetables, chicken soup, and water

Trout baked in coconut cream

Salad of tomato and cucumber

DAY 8

BREAKFAST

Fried egg

Vegetable cutlet

Tea

MIDMORNING SNACK

Cucumber slices

LUNCH

A balanced diet: beans and chicken soup

The perfect roast beef with avocado, lemon, and cream sauce.

Diced mixed salad w/ olive oil dressing

AFTERNOON SNACK

Coconut water

DINNER

Beef and vegetable soup

Little nuggets of chicken with a creamy garlic sauce.

Roasted vegetables with sesame seed oil

DAY 9

BREAKFAST

Toast with cheese and vegetables

Tea

10 AM SNACK

Cucumber slices

LUNCH

Chicken soup is good for the soul

Baked lamb chops with a garlic aioli sauce

Grilled mixed vegetables

AFTERNOON SNACK

Coconut water

DINNER

Cream of beef soup

Baked chicken and salad

.

DAY 10

BREAKFAST

Scrambled eggs with cheese and veggies

Tea

Have your mid morning snack

Cucumber slices

LUNCH

Mixed vegetables and chicken soup

Chicken with grilled vegetables

Mixed salad with sesame seed oil and lemon

AFTERNOON SNACK

Coconut water

DINNER

Beef and vegetables cream soup is a great meal for breakfast.

Healthy steak and healthy vegetables

A green salad with coconut oil and vinegar dressing

DAY 11

BREAKFAST

Fried egg with fried tofu

Grilled mixed vegetables

Tea

Mid-morning snack

Cucumber slices

LUNCH

Mushroom and onion soup

Fried fish with cream cheese and mayo garlic sauce

Have a mixed salad with a mustard sauce

AFTERNOON SNACK

Coconut water

DINNER

Avocado cream soup

Baked chicken with sweet & sour vegetables

Lemon and mint dressing for vegetables

DAY 12

BREAKFAST

Fried sausages and stir-fried vegetables with cream cheese

Tea

Your pre-workout nutrition

Cucumber slices

LUNCH

Clear chicken and vegetable broth

Stir -fried broccoli and chicken

Sliced grilled cucumber with mayonnaise and garlic dressing

AFTERNOON SNACK

Coconut water

DINNER

Perfect for warming up in the winter.

Beef & vegetables with cream cheese and spaghetti squash

Mixed salad, sliced and dressed

DAY 13

BREAKFAST

Egg cooked in pasta and cheese with vegetables

Tea

MID-MORNING SNACK

Cucumber slices

LUNCH

Cream of broccoli soup and chicken soup

Fried prawns with grilled potatoes

Olivier avocado salad

AFTERNOON SNACK

Coconut water

DINNER

Broccoli and tomato soup

A baked salmon with tomato cream sauce and avocado chunks with lemon and olive oil dressing

.

.

DAY 14

BREAKFAST

Hard-boiled egg with cream cheese

Scrambled eggs with fried sausage and vegetables

Tea

MID-MORNING snack

Mixed nuts

LUNCH

Make clear chicken and vegetable broth

Grilled shrimp with vegetables

Diced, fresh salad with your choice of dressing

AFTERNOON SNACK

Strawberries

DINNER

By Beef + Vegetable Soup

Grilled chicken with roasted broccoli and cream cheese sauce

Chopped salad

DIET PLAN FOR THE THIRD WEEK

Atkins diet Phase 2 allows weekly addition of 5 grammes of net carbs. In the third week or the first week of the second phase, you may consume 25 grammes of net carbs. Nuts and seeds can be added to the mix one ounce at a time or in a handful. You can start with one ounce of nuts or seeds (sunflower seeds or pumpkin seeds). It's also a good idea to eat an additional half to one-third cup of raspberries or strawberries in addition to the food permitted in Phase 1.

.

•

THIRTEENth DAY

BREAKFAST

Baked eggs, carrots, and sausages are served with a cream sauce.

Tea

METABOLIC Snack for the Middle of the Morning

Seeds from sunflowers

LUNCH

Vegetable-based mutton broth

Chicken kebabs with cream cheese and mayonnaise sauce and veggies

Avocado, lettuce, with lemon and olive oil dressing on a salad.

Snacks during the afternoon

Raspberries

DINNER

Soup with cream of chicken and broccoli

Lemon-marinated swordfish on the grill

Tossed salad with sesame oil and vinegar and shredded vegetables

.

In the sixteenth day of the year.

BREAKFAST

An omelette with cheese and veggies in the colour of the rainbow

Tea

AN INTENSIVE SNACK FOR MIDDAY

Nuts that are mixed together

LUNCH

Chicken and vegetable broth in a clear container

Sautéed bell peppers and onions with barbecued chicken

Salad with iceberg lettuce, cucumber, and dressing

Snacks during the afternoon

Strawberries

DINNER

Broth made from meat and vegetables, crystal clear.

Cream cheese-topped baked chicken with stir-fried veggies.

Dressed with lemon and olive oil, this salad is light and refreshing.

17th day

BREAKFAST

roasted veggie and cheese omelette

Tea

AN INTENSIVE SNACK FOR MIDDAY

Seed mixture

LUNCH

Soup base made from meat and vegetables.

Roast chicken with peanut butter-sautéed veggies

dressing of one's choosing over fresh diced salad

Snacks during the afternoon

Raspberries

DINNER

Soup base made from meat and vegetables.

Coconut cream and lemon sauce on fried fish

Avocados with cherry tomatoes on a bed of lettuce.

THIRTEENTH DAY

BREAKFAST

a boiled egg that is not overcooked

Vegetables and cheese are added to fried sausages.

Tea

AN INTENSIVE SNACK FOR MIDDAY

Nuts that are mixed together

LUNCH

Broth made from vegetables and meat that is clear to the palate

Lemon cheese sauce atop grilled mutton chops with roasted mixed veggies

Avocado, tomato, fresh sliced cucumbers and shredded lettuce

Snacks during the afternoon

Strawberries

DINNER

Clear broth made with chicken and vegetables

Kebabs of meat, greens, and stir-fried veggies barbecued on the grill

Fresh diced mixed salad with vinegar and olive oil dressing

The 19th day of the year

BREAKFAST

Eggs, cheese, veggies, and sausages in a scrambled egg dish

Tea

AN INTENSIVE SNACK FOR MIDDAY

Seed mixture

LUNCH

Boiling water made from pure vegetables.

Vegetables grilled with grilled beef

Lemon and sesame seed oil in a fresh salad toss

Snacks during the afternoon

Raspberries

DINNER

Clear meat and vegetable stock.

Cherry tomato and cucumber salad on the side of the fried fish

It's Day 20 today.

BREAKFAST

Vegetable and cream cheese omelette

Tea with fried sausages

AN INTENSIVE SNACK FOR MIDDAY

Nuts that are mixed together

LUNCH

Clear broth made with chicken and vegetables

Braised mutton with vegetables

Slicing an avocado fresh from the tree

Snacks during the afternoon

Strawberries

DINNER

Clear meat and vegetable stock.

Mixed veggies sautéed in a cream cheese sauce with roasted beef

a salad of sliced cucumbers, lettuce, and tomatoes

TWENTY-NINTH DAY

BREAKFAST

Eggs, cheese, and veggies in a scramble.

Sausages fried to a crisp

Tea

AN INTENSIVE SNACK FOR MIDDAY

Seed mixture

LUNCH

Soup with chicken and vegetables in a cream base

Roasted chicken and mixed veggies in a baking dish

Squeezed lemon juice over avocados and olives.

Snacks during the afternoon

Strawberries

DINNER

a creamy soup made with beef and vegetables

Steak and roasted veggies in a brown sauce

Yogurt

This is the second phase of the diet plan, which is the fourth week.

Unsweetened and unflavored yoghurt can now be added to the weekly allowance.

•

•

•

•

•

•

DAY 22

BREAKFAST

Omelette with cheese

Stir-fried veggies and tofu served with a fried crust

Sausage that has been deep-fried.

Tea

AN INTENSIVE SNACK FOR MIDDAY

Nuts that are mixed together

LUNCH

Chicken, onion, and mushroom soup

Vegetables cooked in cream sauce with grilled chicken cutlets

Yogurt

Snacks during the afternoon

Raspberries

DINNER

Cream soup with beef and assorted veggies

Kebabs of beef and veggies

chopped cucumber and lettuce from the refrigerator or garden

The 23rd day

BREAKFAST

Sauteed mixed veggies and a fried egg

Sausage on the grill

Tea

AN INTENSIVE SNACK FOR MIDDAY

Seed mixture

LUNCH

Broth made from vegetables and meat that is clear to the palate

Roasted chicken and veggies in a crockpot

Yogurt

Snacks during the afternoon

Strawberries

DINNER

Tofu with Cream of Mutton and Vegetables

Cream cheese sauce over roasted meat and baked veggies.

Olives with cherry tomatoes are a delicious combination.

THIRTEENTH DAY

BREAKFAST

Eggs, boiled or fried

Mixture of grilled veggies

Cream cheese with fried sausage.

Tea

AN INTENSIVE SNACK FOR MIDDAY

Nuts that are mixed together

LUNCH

Broth made from vegetables and meat that is clear to the palate

Peanut butter encrusted meatballs and grilled veggies

Yogurt

Snacks during the afternoon

Raspberries

DINNER

a creamy soup made with beef and vegetables

Prepared with grilled fish and veggies; served with a fresh tossed salad.

JOURNAL NUMBER 25

BREAKFAST

Vegetable omelette with cheese

Sausage that has been deep-fried.

Tea

AN INTENSIVE SNACK FOR MIDDAY

Seed mixture

LUNCH

Broth made from vegetables and meat that is clear to the palate

Coconut cream and lemon sauce baked fish and veggies

Yogurt

Snacks during the afternoon

Strawberries

DINNER

Chicken and vegetable broth in a clear container

Kebabs of marinated meat served with a side of grilled veggies

Avo on the half-cut

TWENTY-SIXH DAY

BREAKFAST

Veggies and tofu scrambled eggs with cheese

Sausage that has been deep-fried.

Tea

AN INTENSIVE SNACK FOR MIDDAY

Nuts that are mixed together

LUNCH

Clear mutton and vegetable broth

grilled chicken breast with sour cream sauce and grilled veggies Yogurt

Snacks during the afternoon

Raspberries

DINNER

Broth made from vegetables and meat that is clear to the palate

Roasted carrots, fried mutton chops, and gravy

Cucumber slices with cherry tomatoes

DATE OF THE 27TH DAY

BREAKFAST

Tofu, cheese, and veggies in a baked egg bake

Sausage on the grill

Tea

AN INTENSIVE SNACK FOR MIDDAY

Seed mixture

LUNCH

The broth is made from meat and veggies.

With grilled mixed veggies, fried chicken wings

Yogurt

Snacks during the afternoon

Strawberries

DINNER

Clear mutton and vegetable broth

Steak and roasted veggies in a brown sauce

Avo on the half-cut

28th day

BREAKFAST

With cheese and veggies, an omelette

Sausage on the grill

Tea

AN INTENSIVE SNACK FOR MIDDAY

Nuts that are mixed together

LUNCH

Chicken and vegetable broth in a clear container

Grilled mixed veggies and baked fish

Yogurt

Snacks during the afternoon

Raspberries

DINNER

Broth made from vegetables and meat that is clear to the palate

Grilled veggies accompany a steak of beef.

Cucumbers and lettuce chopped.

Safety and efficacy of Atkins diet T The Atkins diet encourages the use of fat reserves in the body, rather than carbohydrates as a source of fuel for the body.

energy sources To compensate for the loss of energy provided by carbs, our systems begin to break down stored body fats for energy.

Proteins, lipids, and carbs are all sources of energy for the human body. macronutrients, or the building blocks of our food, are also referred to as fuels for the body. Carbohydrates are necessary for the body to convert from storing fat to storing energy. Adipose or fatty tissue can only be broken down if carbs are eliminated from the diet, hence a dramatic reduction in carbohydrates is essential to lose weight.

Long-term adherence to the Atkins diet might be difficult. Numerous research have been conducted in an effort to better understand the benefits and drawbacks of the Atkins diet. Many studies have shown that the diet helps people lose weight and lower their cholesterol and triglycerides in their blood. The Atkins Nutritional Approach not only helps you lose weight, but it also changes the way you eat for the better. In addition to boosting energy and improving health conditions, the diet can also help to reduce one's weight.

Patients with diabetes, heart disease, renal disease, or other medical conditions should speak with their doctor before beginning this diet to ensure that it is safe for them to follow. The fundamental goal of this diet is to ensure that all of the food's energy sources are being used equally. No trimming of meat or avoiding fats and oils are required in order to follow this diet.

One of the most common causes of ill health is believed to be a diet heavy in carbohydrates, such as sugar, refined flour, and other carbohydrate-rich dietary items. When it comes to a certain diet, there may be a few differences between the old and new versions. Because the body is attempting to acclimatise to the new dietary patterns it is experiencing throughout the induction period, it is not recommended that you exercise during this time. Adding a workout plan to your diet should be postponed for at least two weeks before beginning.

As a result of the diet's high fat and protein composition in the past, medical authorities questioned its overall safety. Our bodies immediately shift to a higher intake of fat and protein when we decrease our carbohydrate consumption. We call them macronutrients because they are the only three nutrients that provide us with energy and make up the bulk of our meals. The Atkins diet advocates for ensuring that its adherents are well-nourished while maintaining a sense of well-being. First, 20 grammes of net carbs per day are allowed, then 5 grammes per week for the second phase, then 10 grammes per week for phase three.

Before entering ketosis, the body expends all of its glycogen reserves in the form of glycogen. In the absence of one of these nutrients, the others will begin to produce energy to compensate.

Fats, carbs, and proteins are all energy-producing nutrients. Fat is the primary storage form for excess amounts of these nutrients. Starvation or fasting causes the body to adapt and use alternative forms of energy, such as fats and proteins, as a source of fuel. Ketone bodies, which are the principal source of energy for the brain, are the result of fat breakdown and usage.

As much as one fifth of our overall energy usage comes from the brain alone. The brain consumes far more energy than any other organ in the body, owing to its high fat content. In the absence of glucose, the brain will adapt to use ketones as a source of energy. Is ketosis abnormal? No, it's just the body's natural response to low carbohydrate intake.

There are times when there are no carbs available and our bodies must use fat as a source of energy. Weight loss can be achieved by incorporating more fats into our diet, which promote fat catabolism. The Atkins plan does not need you to completely cut out carbs from your diet, but rather to gradually reintroduce them back into your system over a period of time. Many studies have shown that this diet can lower LDL (bad) cholesterol while raising HDL (good) cholesterol, which is a surprising finding.

There is also worry that this diet is overly heavy in protein, which might cause renal damage as a result. The presence of ketone bodies in the body, it is hypothesised, may also contribute to foul breath caused by the diet. Nausea, a fruity breath odour, and a lack of appetite are all possible adverse symptoms of ketosis. Additionally, many people are unable to afford a high-protein diet because of budgetary restraints.

Short-term weight reduction has been reported by some of those who have tried this diet, while others have had difficulty achieving the desired outcomes because of lapses in consistency. This diet should not be followed when pregnant or nursing. Since its high fat content has been linked to cardiovascular illness, there has been a lot of worry about its safety. If you follow it for a long length of time, your chances of acquiring a heart-related condition may increase.

Saturated fat intake should be kept to a minimum under all circumstances. If you wish to stick to the Atkins diet for a long length of time, it is imperative that you incorporate healthy fats and oils into your diet. Exercise, in addition to a healthy diet, can be included in the second phase to assist prevent muscle loss and promote muscle gain.

The kidneys may be overworked to eliminate toxicity if they have to work harder to remove ketones produced in excess. In addition to constipation and diarrhoea, following this diet might cause a deficiency or excess of fibre.

For low-carbohydrate diets, you don't have to give up your morning meal. A low-carb Atkins breakfast may satisfy your yearning for a griddle- or oven-fresh meal, and help you start your day off guilt-free and refreshed.

In only three minutes, you can have a coconut and almond muffin.

The only way to acquire a muffin in under three minutes is to buy one from the store, but this recipe proves you incorrect.

Ingredients:

2 tablespoons of almond meal

3 tablespoons of high-fiber coconut flour

1 teaspoon of artificial sweetener (sucralose based)

Baking powder, 14 teaspoon

0.5 tsp. of cinnamon

1/8 teaspoon of salt

The yolk of one egg (large)

1 tablespoon of extra virgin olive oil

Directions:

Add the ingredients to a coffee cup and stir. Mix together.

Add the oil and the egg, and mix well. Stir until the mixture is completely incorporated.

3) Microwave on high for 60 seconds. 4) Using a knife, remove from cup, slice, spread with desired topping, and enjoy!

Waffles from Belgium

Here's a low-carb method to have a scrumptious griddle-cooked supper.

Ingredients:

1 cup soy flour made from whole grains

1/2 cup granulated sweetener (sucralose based)

3-teaspoon powdered baking soda

SALT, 1/2 TSP

14 cup heavy cream

a total of three eggs (large)

1-tablespoon sugar-free agave nectar

A quarter of a cup

Directions:

1. Preheat the waffle iron. Soy flour, salt, sugar replacement, and baking soda are all combined in a bowl. Stir in the other ingredients (eggs, cream, syrup) until the batter is firm. Add one tablespoon of cold water at a time to the batter until it is spreadable.

Use a nonstick spray to coat the waffle iron before using it. Make a little mound of the batter in the middle of the iron. Cook for a few minutes until crisp and golden. This can be done as many times as necessary until the batter has been used up. Serve it hot.

RECIPES FOR THE HOURLY MEAL

Do you ever become tired in the middle of the day? That's not a problem that can't be solved with a low-carb meal. The following are some delicious recipes to help you get started:

The remainder of the day was spent rejuvenated and refuelled.

Squares of Artichoke with Cheddar Cheese

These low-carb cheese cubes are perfect for packing in your lunchbox. Ingredients:

Extra-virgin olive oil in two tablespoons

3 medium scallions, sliced thinly

3 cloves of garlic

1 box of uncooked frozen artichokes

A quarter teaspoon of oregano

1/4 tsp. red pepper flakes crushed

a total of four eggs (large, whole)

a half cup of Monterey jack (shredded)

All-purpose flour made from whole wheat and soy beans

The two tablespoons of parsley

SALT, 1/2 TSP

A quarter teaspoon of ground black pepper

Directions:

Start by preheating the oven to 325°F.

2. In a medium pan, heat oil and cook scallions until tender. For around 30 seconds more, add the garlic and cook for a further 30 seconds. Pour in the artichokes and simmer until they are cooked through, then add oregano and pepper flakes (about 2 mins.) For approximately five minutes, let the food to cool down a bit.

Using an electric mixer or by hand, blend the soy flour and eggs in a large basin until they are thoroughly mixed. Stir in the artichoke mixture.

Set and golden on top, bake for 30 minutes in an 8" square baking dish, then remove. Cut into squares when cool.

Salad of chicken and pesto

On a sunny afternoon, this quick and easy salad is a great way to get your protein fix.

Ingredients:

An onion, cut into thirds

a half-pound of boneless, skinless chicken breast

1 celery stalk

a third of a cup of mayo

Garlic, salt, and pepper to taste

2 tbsp pesto dressing

Salt in the amount of 1/4 teaspoon

peppercorns, about one-eighth teaspoon

Directions:

A dish of celery and chicken salad with onions and mayonnaise is ready to serve. Place on a bed of fresh, sliced or cherry tomatoes and serve right away. For a maximum of three days, food stored in an airtight container can be kept in the refrigerator.

Salad Ingredients and Vegetable Puree: Fried Chicken

Make a puree out of 1 cup of mixed veggies from the approved list.

2 squeezes of fresh lime

6 thinly chopped garlic cloves

2 tbsps of a cream cheese

A quarter cup of sesame oil

according on your personal preference, add salt and pepper. 1 4-5 ounce chicken quarter

ginger-garlic paste, 1 tbsp

1/4 tsp. ground mustard

Green chile paste, 1 tablespoon For deep frying, add 1/2 tsp paprika, q tbsp apple cider vinegar, and olive oil.

Directions:

Fried garlic in sesame seed oil till golden brown.

Then, add the cream cheese and lemon juice to the pureed veggies and combine thoroughly.

Add salt and pepper to taste, and then combine thoroughly..

Marinade the chicken and other ingredients, save for the oil, for a while before cooking.

Alternatively, you may deep fry the chicken or bake it in an oven that has been preheated.

Sliced avocados, cucumbers, and lettuce are all great accompaniments to the chicken.

8

Recipes for a good meal

You don't need a frozen food tray to have a substantial meal. There are several wonderful, low-carb Atkins-friendly dishes out there that you can create ahead of time and enjoy when you get home from work.

A Maple Mustard Glazed Salmon Omega-3s and proteins abound in this spicy-sweet dish.

Ingredients:

2 tablespoons of sugar-free maple syrup

12 cup of plain old city water

3 tbsps Mustard from Dijon, France

2 garlic cloves

Salt in a pinch

Wild Atlantic salmon weighing 2 lbs.

Directions:

Melt butter in a small saucepan over medium heat. Add other ingredients and boil until reduced to about half a cup. Cool.

Set broiler to medium-high. Place fish on rack of greased broiler pan, skin side down. Add a pinch of salt to taste. For six minutes, broil 4 inches from the flame.

Braai for another 4 minutes, brushing with sauce and checking for doneness.

Pork Roasted with Ginger and Cranberry

This is a low-carb dish that's perfect for the holidays because it's sweet but not overpowering.

Ingredients:

For four pounds of bone-in, center-ribbed pork chops or roast

Adobo sauce with chipotle chiles (1 each)

1 cup chopped cranberries

syrup of your choice, 2 ounces of it

a pinch of ginger

SALT, 1/2 TSP

A quarter teaspoon of ground black pepper

Boiling water, chicken broth or consomme

0.5 oz of water

A quarter teaspoon of guar gum.

The butter should be unsalted.

Directions:

1. Heat 12 cup of oil in a large pan over medium heat. Roast is ready to go into the skillet after being seasoned with black pepper and salt to taste. Each side should be browned for about a minute, for a total of four minutes. Set aside to chill.

Chop the cranberries and dice the chipotle pepper.

Salt, pepper, and shredded ginger should be added to the chipotle mixture. Place the leftover mixture in the bottom of a slow cooker and rub it into the meat.

Add cranberries and chicken broth to the edge of the pan, and then stir everything together. Rinsing the roast will remove the rub, so avoid doing so.

Cover and cook for 8 to 10 hours on low heat..

Remove the roast and place it on a serving platter under a tent of aluminium foil, reserving the juices for later. In a slow cooker, add water and guar gum and stir until a thick paste forms. Cook until the sauce thickens, stirring occasionally, over low heat. Season with salt and pepper to taste and add butter to sauce. Serve the roast with the sauce on top.

This dish includes grilled fish, vegetables, and a salad.

Ingredients:

5 ounces of your favourite boneless fish fillet.

1 tbsp. minced garlic

2 squeezes of fresh lime a tablespoon of Worcestershire sauce according on your personal preference, add salt and pepper.

1 cup of diced veggies from the permitted list of vegetables.

2 cloves of garlic, minced

1 tsp of oregano Season to taste with salt and pepper 4 tbsp of sesame seed oil

Directions:

The fish should be marinated in garlic paste, lemon juice, Worcestershire sauce and salt & pepper for a while before cooking.

2. Heat a grill pan and cook the fish until it is done on both sides.

3. Brown the cumin seeds in the oil.

Make sure everything is mixed well before serving.

Stir cook for a few more minutes.

As an accompaniment, serve a fresh salad of your choosing with the fish fillets.

9

Recipes for Snacks

T

It's crucial to keep hunger at bay in order to prevent overeating during meals when dieting. Snacks are a terrific way to keep hunger at bay, and there are many tasty, low-sugar, and low-carbohydrate alternatives.

Baked Brie with Sun Dried Tomatoes and Pine Nuts Ingredients:

8 ounces of brie

Sun-dried tomatoes in a tbsp

1 tbsp. parsley

Pine nuts in half an ounce (dried)

Directions:

Set the oven temperature to 450 degrees.

Remove cheese's rind with a sharp knife and set it in a pie dish.

Spread the parsley and sun-dried tomato mixture evenly over the cheese. Add the pine nuts and bake for a further ten minutes, or until they are toasted and fragrant.

Ingredients for Cauliflower Buffalo Hot Wings:

1 cauliflower head (large)

Oil of choice: 2 tbsps

4 tbsp. of red spicy wing sauce.

Unsalted butter, about two tablespoons

There should be 3 TBSp of siracha chilli sauce in this dish.

The equivalent of one-and-a-half pounds of roquefort

Directions:

Preheat the oven to 375°F.

Add one tablespoon of olive oil to the cauliflower and chop into tiny florets. Roast for 35 to 40 minutes, until the meat is fork-tender.

Add siracha and spicy wing sauce to small sauce pan while cauliflower roasts; let simmer for a few minutes. Serve at room temperature with a drizzle of melted butter. In a large sauté pan, heat the remaining oil. Toss in the cauliflower and cook for one more minute, tossing it until it is well-coated with hot sauce. Serve immediately with a generous sprinkling of cheese.

Guacamole with Cucumbers

Ingredients:

1/4 of a cup of cukes (peel on)

A single jalapeo pepper.

Red onions, 1/16 cup (chopped)

1/8 tsp. garlic

Cilantro is 1/4 cup.

One fruit of the tree: an avocado

1 tablespoon of lime juice

a cup and a half of chilli powder

Directions:

Cucumber, red onion, and jalapeno, all diced finely, should be chopped into 1/4-inch pieces. Set aside chopped cilantro and minced garlic.

2. In a bowl, mash the avocado with a fork. Use as much or as little of each of the following: salt, black pepper, and lime juice according to taste.

Garlic, onion, cucumber and cilantro are all excellent additions. Combine the ingredients and revel in the results.

Recommendations for Dessert Recipes

Having a low blood sugar does not necessitate giving up dessert. Many sugar-free options are available to satisfy your sweet taste.

choices that allow you to have your cake and eat it too.

Custard ice cream is made up of the following:

3 mugs of thick whipping cream

The yolks of three eggs (large)

Egg, entire (large)

34 of a sugar alternative (sucralose based)

SALT, 1/8 TSP

Vanilla extract in half a teaspoon

Directions:

1. Bring cream to a boil in a large saucepan over medium heat. Egg, yolk, salt and sugar replacement should be whisked together while the cream is cooking.

In a separate bowl, beat the eggs with the cream and then return the mixture to the pan. Mixture should thicken enough to coat a spoon after 1 to 2 minutes of stirring on a medium-low temperature.

Pour into a separate basin and allow to cool. Add a dash of vanilla to it.

Refrigerate for about 4 hours, until cooled, with plastic wrap over the surface. Serve immediately after freezing.

Frozen Cheesecake Balls with Peanut Butter and Chocolate:

6 oz. of sour cream

Nutella (naturally roasted) in a cup 33% less sugar and sodium

A teaspoon of xylitol

vanilla essence, about a teaspoonful

Stevia leaf, if you'd like.

Heavy cream, one cup

Zanthan gum: 1/8th teaspoon

Three chocolate bars with salted caramel and extra crunch crunch

Directions:

To make xylitol powder, place 2 tablespoons in a blender and process 3-4 times until it is pulverised.

Using a mixer on medium speed, blend softened cream cheese until it is creamy. Substitute powdered sugar for the white stuff. A symphony of sound Add a sprinkle of stevia for extra sweetness if desired.

Two tablespoons xanthan gum are added to 1 cup of cream and the mixture is whipped until frothy.

3. Slice snack bars in half, then finely chop them and add them to the mix. Form a ball with a 2 tablespoon scoop and place it on a wax paper-covered baking sheet. Once frozen, remove from freezer and store for at least 4 hours in the refrigerator. 30 minutes before serving, let partly thawed food sit in refrigerator. This recipe should make enough for 24 balls.

Brownies with Chocolate Syrup Ingredients:

heavy cream, 3 tablespoons.

4 ounces baking chocolate, unsweetened

An 8 tbsp. portion of unsalted butter

Powdered erythritol

1 Stevia packet

1 cup heavy cream 2 tablespoons sugar 1 teaspoon vanilla extract

Eggs from four hens (large)

2/3 of a cup

2 tablespoons of chocolate syrup

2 lbs. of almond meal

3-teaspoon powdered baking soda

The salt content is equal to one teaspoon

Directions:

Preheat the oven to 350 degrees Fahrenheit and grease a 9-by-2-by-13-inch baking sheet. In a microwave-safe dish, combine the heavy cream and chocolate and heat for 20-second intervals. Set aside to chill.

2. Cream Melt the 1 1/2 cups of erythritol and butter together until frothy using a mixer on medium speed for about five minutes. Add vanilla extract and stevia. Blend for 30 seconds after each addition of an egg. Then add the completely cooled chocolate mixture and beat until well-combined. Add the water and continue beating for another minute.

In a small bowl, combine almond flour, baking powder, salt, and cocoa powder. Then mix for a few seconds until the mixture is thoroughly incorporated into the eggs. A toothpick may be placed into the centre of the cake and come out clean after 30 minutes of baking. Serve when it has cooled. For a maximum of five days, store in the refrigerator.

Chapter Three

DRINK RECIPES

Coffee, smoothies, or something with a little kick are all low-carb options for adding your favourite beverage to your diet without guilt.

Ingredients for a coffee slushie:

One and one-half ounces of sugar-free vanilla syrup

decaffeinated coffee, 2 ounces

2 teaspoons of vanilla whey

Vanilla whey protein isolate

Heavily-creamed milk

2 cubes of ice

Directions:

2. Put the ice cubes into a blender and pulverise them. Pour in the coffee, protein powder mix, and syrup.

2. Blend until smooth on high. Make a creamy sauce by whisking up with heavy cream. Blend together until smooth.

Smoothie with Blackberries:

A quarter-cup of blackberries, thawed

Coconut milk in its unsweetened form (almond or soy milk may be substituted)

1 ounce of vanilla whey protein isolate

Organic whole golden flaxseed meal, 1 tsp.

cinnamon, 14 tsp

Ground allspice into a powder

Vanilla extract in half a teaspoon

Directions:

Blend the frozen blackberries with the protein powder, vanilla, milk, and spices in a food processor until smooth. Blend together until smooth.

Citrus and Lime Margherita

Ingredients:

Lime juice with half a lime

1 tbsp of sugar-free syrup (sucralose based)

Six ounces of tequila 1 orange fluid ounce

An orange juice concentrate of 1 fluid ounce

Directions:

1. Juice and zest limes. Blend the sugar substitute and lime zest in a blender until they're finely

ground. Serve with lime and orange wedges on the side for garnish.

Garnish with lime wedges before serving in cocktail glasses.

12

Diabetic management with the ATKINS DIET

The high consumption of refined carbohydrates in the typical American diet is one of the primary causes of the epidemic of type 2 diabetes in our country. American grocery aisles remain dominated by white flour, sugar, and other items with a high glycemic index, despite a growing trend toward a healthy lifestyle. In order to get rid of the extra insulin, your pancreas goes into an emergency mode when you eat meals that are high in glucose.

After a certain point in one's adulthood, the symptoms of this excess of sugar begin to appear and one's weight begins to rise. These signs and symptoms can be seen in the majority of obese persons who follow a high-carb diet.

Insulin resistance affects a huge percentage of the world's obese population. An abnormally high quantity of insulin is produced by the pancreas in response to an abnormally low level of insulin in the body, causing blood sugar levels to plunge to dangerously low levels. The body may release adrenaline in an effort to bring the blood sugar level back to normal, which might lead to further issues.

The first three stages of diabetes 1 are seldom diagnosed. Insulin, which produces a lot of fat, means that by the time someone is diagnosed with diabetes, they are probably already overweight or obese. As a result, their pancreas is already fatigued, and their blood sugar levels are constantly fluctuating, leading to full-blown diabetes.

Diabetes imposes restrictions and causes discomfort on one's life. In stage 5 diabetes, when insulin levels are exceedingly low, you may begin to lose weight because your blood sugar levels are so high that insulin can no longer control them. As a result of excessive urine, your body begins to burn anything it can in order to power itself. This results in persistent thirst.

As a result of Atkins,

Several recent studies have shown that a low-carbohydrate diet helps improve glucose and fat lipid management in patients with type 2 diabetes. Compared to a group of people on a high carb diet, those on a low fat diet had substantial improvements in weight loss, blood sugar management, and medication reduction as compared to those on a high carb diet. Managing type 2 diabetes requires a lot of weight reduction, however many of the drugs given for diabetic therapy can cause weight gain. If you're looking for an alternative to medicine, a low-carb diet can help you lose weight while also keeping your blood sugar levels in check.

Medication-Induced Obesity

In order to effectively manage diabetes, one must do much more than simply reduce blood glucose levels. Having insulin resistance as a sign of type 2 diabetes indicates that the glucose will resist insulin's efforts to control it. This means that our most powerful weapon against it, insulin, may not be able to get through to our bodies, resulting in a high dose of insulin for most diabetics, which can lead to weight gain as a result. Alternative drugs have been created, however weight gain is almost always the outcome of attempting to manage blood glucose aggressively.

Medication-induced hypoglycemia

Hypoglycemia, which causes symptoms such as shakiness, weariness, and disorientation, can also occur as a side effect of blood sugar control efforts. To alleviate these sensations, people often turn to sugary foods, which boost their blood sugar and restart the cycle of high glucose levels. After completing the first few weeks of the Atkins regimen, many type 2 patients seldom encounter hypoglycemia because they work with their primary care physicians to alter their medicines.

Reducing Calories Isn't Enough.

While cutting back on calories may seem like a simple way to cure and avoid the symptoms of type 2 diabetes, weight loss isn't always enough to merit the discontinuation of medication if the carbohydrate consumption continues to rise. Also, because diabetes medications can produce an increase in hunger, it may be difficult for a diabetic to lose weight.

Type 2 diabetes can be well managed by the Atkins Diet, which eliminates sugar and reduces overall carb consumption. Stabilizing blood glucose levels while reducing the need for diabetic medication is made possible by limiting carbohydrate consumption to animal proteins and basic vegetables.

Diabetics should eat a low-carb diet

A low-carbohydrate diet is commonly suggested for people with type 2 diabetes since insulin resistance is a direct result of ingesting too many carbohydrates. If you feel that your type 2 diabetes is caused by consuming too many carbs, the following suggestions may be helpful to you:

1. Make use of a carb counter. Keeping track of how many carbohydrates you eat is an excellent strategy to protect yourself from overindulging.

2. Consume vegetables that do not include starch. Choose vegetables that come in a spectrum of hues. Vegetables with low glycemic indices, such as cauliflower, asparagus, eggplant and broccoli, are good for a low-carb diet.

3. Eat a lot of whole grain. A diabetic diet must include plenty of fruits, vegetables, and other high-fiber foods.

Stay away from sugars. Sugar and high-fructose corn syrup-laden foods can raise blood sugar levels, which can lead to weight gain and obesity. If you're hankering for something sweet, consider sugarless desserts.

5. Have a Good Morning Meal! As crucial as ever as a meal for your body and brain! A healthy blood sugar balance is maintained by eating a nutritious breakfast every day. Breakfast is the most important meal of the day. At least three meals and two snacks a day are necessary.

Don't be scared of fats. Natural and mono-saturated fats, such as those found in olive oil, can decrease cholesterol and are an essential element of a balanced low-carb diet.

Ingredients: 1. Cheddar Omelet with Sauteed Tomatoes and Zucchini

Oil: 1 tbsp.

Half a cup of shredded zucchini

Tomatoes, half a medium

2 big eggs, entire

1/2 cup of shredded cheddar cheese

Directions:

In a pan, heat the olive oil over medium-high heat. Add the zucchini and cook until it is soft (about 2-3 minutes). Cook the tomatoes for one minute after they have been added to the pot. Afterwards, remove the skillet from the stovetop.

Pour the beaten eggs into the skillet and cook for a few minutes. It should only take a couple of minutes for bubbles to develop and the bottom edges to start to solidify. Flip the omelette by delicately lifting one of the edges. Cook for an additional two minutes.

3. Top with zucchini and tomatoes, then half the cheese and half the egg mixture. Add the rest

of the cheese. Remove one side of the omelette from the pan and place it on top of the melted cheese and veggie mixture. Cook until the cheese begins to melt, about one minute. Put the remainder of the veggies on top and take it off the heat. You may eat this for both breakfast and lunch.

2. Asparagus and Leek Soup (4 servings) Ingredients:

Unsalted butter: two teaspoons

A single leek, sliced thinly

3/4 lb. of asparagus

1 tsp of minced fresh garlic

1.15 ounces of chicken broth or bouillon in a can

heavy cream, 3 tablespoons.

Directions:

1. In a large saucepan, melt the butter over medium heat. Add the leeks and cook for 3 minutes more. After one more minute, add the asparagus and cook for a final time. Add the garlic and cook for a further 30 seconds.

Bring the broth to a boil in the meantime.

Simmer for 8-10 minutes or until asparagus is tender, then remove lid and reduce heat to low.

Incorporate cream and seasonings, like salt, pepper, and peppercorns. Using a blender or food processor, puree the ingredients until they are completely smooth.

It is best to re-heat any leftovers before serving. Salt and pepper to taste using freshly ground black pepper. A delicious way to start your dinner or to round off your meal.

Ingredients for Chocolate Coconut Truffles:

Heavy cream is 3/4 cup.

Sugar replacement based on sucralose: 2 tbsp.

butter, unsalted, about two tablespoons

chocolate chips sugar free, 14 ounces

3 ounces of baking chocolate that is not sweetened

2/3 cup heavy whipping cream

4 oz. of coconut (dried)

Raw cashews, two servings (organic)

Directions:

In a small saucepan, combine the butter, cream, and sugar substitute. Let it stew for a while. Pour the hot cream mixture over the chopped baking chocolate and let it sit for five minutes.

Stir until the chocolate is fully melted. Add 1/2 cup coconut and vanilla essence to the mixture. Stir occasionally while refrigerating for about 1 hour and 45 minutes. It will be difficult to form truffles if the mixture is too hard to work with.

3. Toast the remaining 1/2 cup of coconut in a pan over medium heat, stirring often, until it is nicely toasted. Allow to cool in a basin.

In a bowl, combine the ingredients and roll into 32 balls the size of big marbles. Spread toasted coconut on half the balls and cashews on the other half. Store in a well-sealed, airtight container with wax paper between the layers. Refrigeration is recommended for a maximum of one week.

Changing one's body shape

Weight gain isn't just about the amount of it you have, but where it's located. One of the main signs of pre-diabetes or metabolic syndrome is an apple-shaped, or abdominal obesity. These people are also at risk for high blood pressure, increased cholesterol levels in the body and insulin resistance. So, if you have a concentrated kind of obesity, you are more likely to get heart disease and diabetes than someone who is more pear-shaped.

To find out which category you belong to, take a measurement around your midsection. Apple-shaped bodies can be found in both men and women who are over 35 inches tall or over 40 inches tall.

It's more detrimental to your health than fat deposited elsewhere on the body because it contains two forms of fat: subcutaneous and fat around key organs (visceral fat). Viscose fats may release hormones that cause elevated blood lipids and insulin resistance, according to researchers.

Studies have shown that women and men with more abdominal fat are three times more likely to acquire coronary heart disease and three times more likely to develop diabetes than those with less centralised fat distribution.

Maintaining a healthy weight

Even though decreasing weight across your body can help you slim down your midsection, there is no way to specifically pinpoint where the most weight will be lost. It's possible that modest exercise can assist. There were two groups in the 12-month study: one was allocated to 45-minute moderate exercise five days a week; the other was assigned to an hour-long stretching session one week. Both groups were monitored for changes in body mass index (BMI) and waist circumference. To lose weight, neither group went on a diet. Women in the stretching group actually gained visceral fat during the research, whereas those who engaged in moderate exercise shed between 3.4 and 6.9 percent of their visceral fat. Even while the women in the exercise group dropped just a little proportion of their total body weight, the vast majority of it was visceral fat. This suggests that a regular, persistent fitness programme can help reduce abdominal fat, which is a risk factor for diabetes.

Including Atkins in the equation can increase the significance of the results. It's possible to improve your cholesterol levels, lower your blood pressure and increase insulin resistance by following the Atkins diet and exercising regularly. This will help you lose more fat and improve your chances of controlling your type 2 diabetes, which is a complication of the metabolic syndrome.

THE MODERN WORLD OF ATKINS

When you're on the move, in a restaurant, or even at work, you may be presented with alternatives that don't fit the Atkins diet. Breakfast carts are full with donuts, bagels, and danishes, and chances are the menu at your neighbourhood restaurant isn't geared toward accommodating your dietary restrictions. There is no need to worry about any of this because you can always change your diet if the menu does not. A way out can always be found as long as you have the right tactics.

Always Have a Plan B in Mind

In order to avoid being tempted by the office sweets in the conference room, avoid arriving for the meeting hungry. Breakfast with a robust mushroom omelette will give you the strength to resist the temptations of the office. Check out the cafeteria menu if you need to eat on the fly. Please tell me there is something to eat on the table. Make sure you have a healthy choice on hand by brown bagging it.

A Place to Get a Quick Lunch

In general, fast food restaurants have a negative reputation in the health business, but surprisingly, most entree options, including burgers and chicken fingers, are Atkins friendly; it's the extras, however, that you need watch out for It's best to think about what you want to eat ahead of time and avoid ordering extra sides like French fries or onion rings when you see them.

Restaurants

If you eat at a certain restaurant on a frequent basis, the staff is likely to be accommodating to your dietary needs. Let the waiter know that you're on a sugar-free diet and cannot handle any sweeteners.

In this way, you won't have to be concerned about the presence of hidden sugars in the menu options you select.

Avoid thickening your food with breading, sauces, or flour. Carbohydrates may be found in unexpected locations, so be on the lookout. Burgers and fried chicken may contain grains, flour, or bread crumbs.

Don't be afraid to ask the chef directly about the ingredients in a meal. Because you are the one who decides how much to tip the wait staff, they will normally go along with your wishes.

You'll be surprised at how many great restaurants there are in your area that use quality products to create delicious meals. Elegant dinners such as roast beef, duck, lobster, and poached salmon may all be enjoyed without deviating from a strict weight loss plan..

Consider asking for a vegetable tray instead of the bread basket if you find it irresistible. Try to keep the bread basket away from your face if there is another person at the table who wants it.

Parties

In the event that you're attending an ice cream party, you may not discover anything to eat that you like. Let your host know and inquire as to what he or she plans to serve if this is the case. Make sure you have a salad and protein-rich meal before you depart, or carry some food with you if you can't find something suitable.

In and Out of the Kitchen with Atkins

Traveling may be difficult. Traveling, coping with time shifts, and checking into and out of hotels can all disrupt your normal routines, but your nutrition need not be one of them. There are several ways to incorporate the Atkins diet into your travel plans if you're thinking about going on a trip.

Ahead of Schedule

Take a snack with you no matter how you get there: by car, by plane, or by rail. Consider checking ahead to see if there are any low-carb choices on the route. While in the airport, you might want to stop by the salad bar to load up on some veggies and poultry. Whether you're driving or on a train, bring along a bottle of club soda, bottled water, coffee, or herbal tea. If you're on the go,

Atkins bars are an excellent alternative because they're easy to carry.

Eat in or take out

Be specific about what you don't want when ordering room service. Do not order toast or buns with your breakfast or supper. Request that the waiter remove any unwanted goods from the room service cart before he leaves. When you're finished, set the tray outside your door to keep the dog from grazing. Keep your eyes peeled in the bar fridge, which is likely to be a landmine of starchy treats. If you believe this would be a challenge, you may want to give up the fridge's key.

Restaurants renowned for their cuisine

It's difficult to resist trying some of the local delicacies when you're in a location known for its diverse culinary offerings. Breakfast should be a low-carb drink or eggs, and lunch should be a protein-rich salad. This should allow you to savour some of the local cuisine in moderation, though. To avoid heavy sauces and breading, go for a speciality dish.

Moving is the best way to stay active.

There's a good chance you're getting plenty of exercise while on a relaxing vacation. You can get some exercise even if you're stuck in a conference room or a car for long periods of time, but it's a good idea to look for alternatives. If you're staying in a hotel that doesn't offer a gym, pack some nice walking shoes and go for a stroll around the neighbourhood.

On the Go Snacks

The following low-carbohydrate choices are great to have on hand when travelling rather than the usual bag of chips and cookie dough:

Sliced vegetables and cream cheese are a great combination.

String cheese, cubes of cheese, and slices of cheese are all options.

3. Trail mix

Eggs, either deviled or hard boiled

5. Almonds

6. Olives

Mixture of popcorn and nuts, no less!

Turkey jerky or beef jerky, your choice (cured, without sugar)

9. Berries

ten. Peanut butter with celery.

Sugar-free candy and snack cakes are also popular.

Also, don't forget to drink enough of water when driving. Everyone in the car should have their own water bottle. If you know where you're going, you'll know where to stop for a bite to eat or a walk. If you want to avoid feeling ravenous, aim to have a nutritious snack or meal every two to three hours. Ensure that you have enough ice and a cooler to keep chilled products cool by packing snacks like those listed above.

CPSIA information can be obtained
at www.ICGtesting.com
Printed in the USA
LVHW040904240822
726654LV00010B/854